Rooted to RISE in Strength

Be strong & courageous
JOSHUA 1:9

Keep Rising!

P.Leimenstoll

Paola Leimenstoll

ISBN: 978-1-957619-02-6

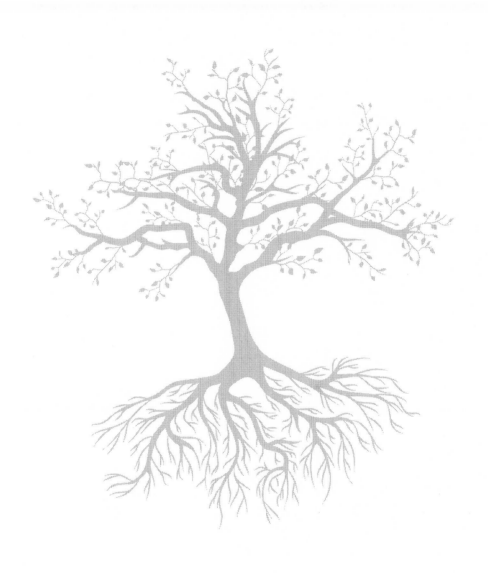

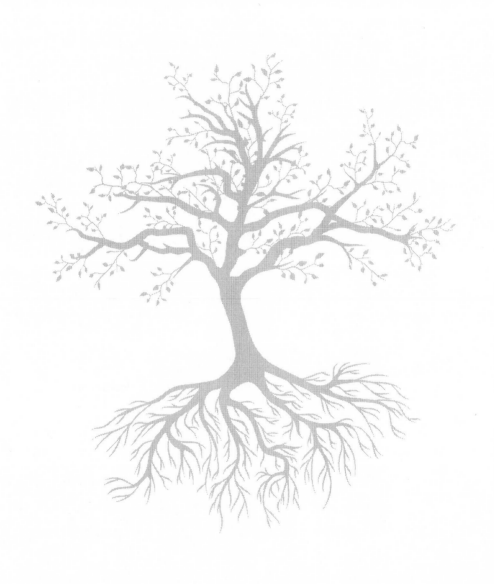

Climbing Mountains

Day 1

"Have I not commanded you? Be strong and courageous, do not be afraid.
Do not be discouraged. For the Lord your God will be with you wherever you go."

- Joshua 1:9

Oh, how I have recited that simple sentence, "Be strong and courageous", throughout my life. But, I truly never understood those words until those were the only words I could cling to. I say cling because life has a funny way of smacking you unexpectedly in the face and having you become discouraged and sometimes afraid. It truly takes courage to step out of your comfort zones. But most importantly, as you start to let go of the comfort you realize just how much stronger you become throughout that process.

I remember when God said, "Hey, I want you to start competing. I want to use you to inspire others who have forgotten who they are, that are lost just like you." I said, "God, you can't be serious . I haven't worn a two piece since I was 17. And hello, remember I am the girl who was diagnosed with an eating disorder at the age of 14." I had all the fears, excuses and reasons why I shouldn't do it.

Well, as you know God got the last laugh. Because in May 2015 I stepped on my first stage, legs shaking and looking at all the other competitors and feeling out of place. I saw the bright lights, the 7 judges and said "God, I showed up but do I truly need to do this?" As my number was called, and I started to walk on the one thing on repeat was: be strong, be courageous. And I felt the chains of body dysmorphia, not good enough, and comparison start to fall away. What replaced it was a calling to help women see that they are truly more than that daily hat they wear.

QUESTION: What does this verse mean to you. Is there one thing holding you back in your comfort zone? _____

_____

_____

_____

_____

_____

_____

_____

_____

_____

_____

_____

_____

_____

_____

_____

_____

_____

_____

_____

_____

_____

_____

_____

PRAYER: Lord, help guide me to be strong and have courage to step out in faith. Guide and direct my path. And remove any fear or discouragement I may have today. Amen

Affirmation to speaking life:

I am strong and courageous!

Song to add to playlist: Warrior - Hannah Kerr

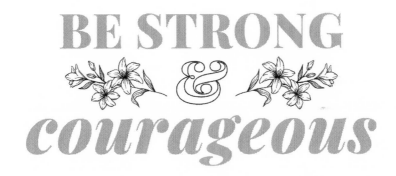

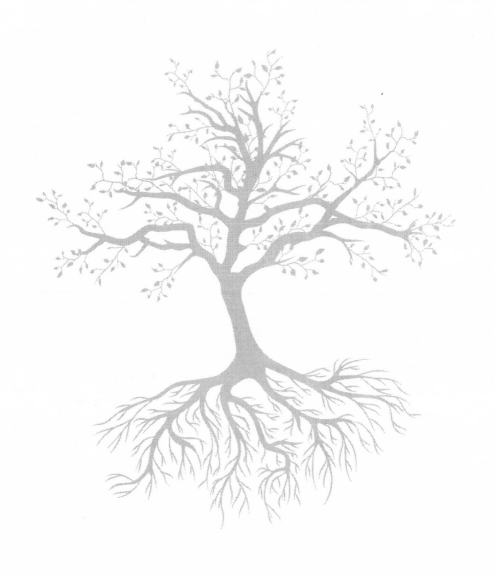

Day 2

Can I not do with you, house of Israel, as this potter does? Declares the lord.
Like clay in the hand of the potter, so are you in my hand.

- Jeremiah 18:6

How amazing is it that no matter the setbacks or trials, you can be renewed, reshaped, recreated and restored?!

2009, was one of the many darkest moments of my life. My marriage was headed to a divorce, and my faith and relationship with God was on the rocks. By day, I was a super mom and by night my best friend was vodka with pineapple. I remember coming home one night and looking my mom in the face and saying if God is so real tell him to show up and show himself. Well, my friends, when you ask God to show up, He does. As I slept, I found myself walking on a path and God showing me a piece of clay so broken , crumbling and had such huge holes. As I watched the potter try to reshape it, I said why doesn't he just toss that away. He looked at me and said, "even though it's so broken it can be restored and become a beautiful masterpiece. You see that clay, Paola? That clay is you and I have great plans for you. You see, I'm about to use you to help others." I started to laugh, use me? I am the biggest train wreck, use me? As we kept watching I witnessed this broken clay start to become something so beautiful. Twelve years later this verse, this moment is the foundation of my brand, and is on the wall of my gym. And even though I look back in wonder. I can say this no matter how broken you feel or what you are going through… you are such a beautiful masterpiece.

QUESTION: Can you look back at a moment in your life where you felt so broken, but you got through? _____

_____

_____

_____

_____

_____

_____

_____

_____

_____

_____

_____

_____

_____

_____

_____

_____

_____

_____

_____

_____

_____

_____

PRAYER: Lord, you know where I'm struggling and sometimes I just feel broken. I ask you Lord that You renew my mind, restore my soul, and reshape me as you remind me how I am a masterpiece. That it is ok to be beautifully broken and that you are forever the potter in my story. Amen

Affirmation to speaking life:

Today I choose to be kind
and to love myself

Song to add to playlist: Beautifully Broken - Plumb

Mindfulness pose: Raised arm pose - hold for 10 repeat for 3

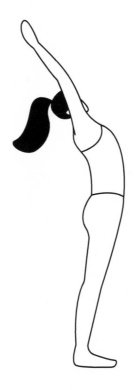

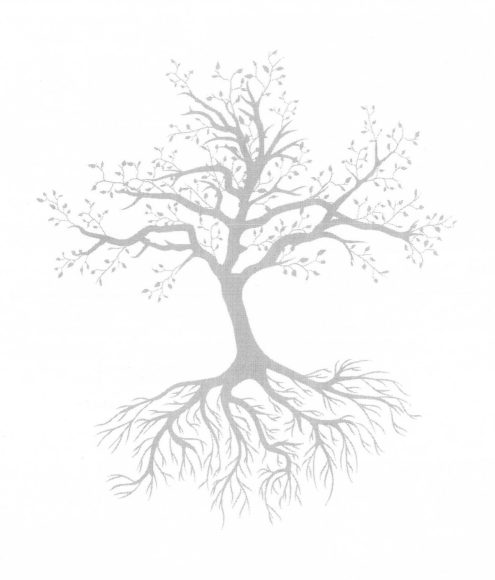

Biting that Tongue

Day 3

As iron sharpens iron, so one person sharpens another.

- Proverbs 27:17

We live in a time where a kind word goes so far. A simple smile spreads so much joy. But, the power of the tongue can either uplift or cause destruction.

There are times, I myself, have caused destruction with this mouth of mine! Sometimes, I am Sophia from the golden girls. I have no filter, speak my mind and sometimes forget that isn't sharpening others.

As a gym owner and trainer, it's continuing to learn whether this speaks life and uplift or is your point more important to be right. And to be honest, let me tell you, as a type 8 enneagram and being Latin, I battle this tongue of mine, because your girl wants to be right. Sometimes, I find myself quoting the Tik Tok video Holy Spirit activate, as I say, "Lord you made me this way." But, then, I am humbled with a gentle reminder. Would you enjoy that being done to you? Is this helping to speak life into people and uplifting and the answer is a simple no.

QUESTION: How can you uplift and speak life into someone today?

_____

_____

_____

_____

_____

_____

_____

_____

_____

_____

_____

_____

_____

_____

_____

_____

_____

_____

_____

_____

_____

_____

_____

PRAYER: Lord help me to speak life into others. Even when I feel like I should be right, help me to give grace. Guide me to encourage others as you encourage me. In your name, Amen .

Affirmation to speaking life:

I choose words that speak life and are full of faith

Song to add to playlist: Speak Life - Toby Mac

Quote: The tongue is but small, soft flesh. Yet it is capable of breaking the strongest bonds and destroying the most powerful relationships. - Yasir Qadhi

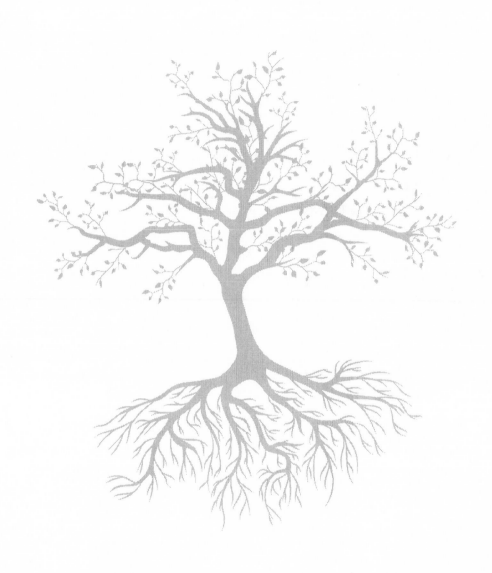

Why Again

Day 4

Don't be afraid; you are worth more than many sparrows.

- Luke 12:7

Life comes at us so hard and things happen where you are asking why? Why is this happening to me? What did I do to make this happen? Once you start down that path, your failures, disappointments, setbacks , and mistakes start to grow. You start to get anxiety and stress and forget one simple thing - who you truly are and it will be ok.

I can look back throughout my life and look at all the moments that I said, "why God, why?" I would breakdown at whatever I was facing and allow stress, fear and anger to take over and sometimes my anxiety would get the best of me. Oh, how many times have I found myself crying and saying I'm done and doubted everything? My favorite line was, "Welp, I screwed up this or this was not meant to be."

But even when those storms come into our lives, the sun always rises. And with that sunrise comes new promises, new hope and most importantly, you are reminded, my sweet friends, how much you are needed. You are so worthy of doing whatever your purpose may be.

QUESTION : Take a minute to look at you. What are three things that you see that remind you of just how worthy you are? _____

_____

_____

_____

_____

_____

_____

_____

_____

_____

_____

_____

_____

_____

_____

_____

_____

_____

_____

_____

_____

_____

_____

_____

PRAYER: Father, thank you for reminding me that even through the storms the sun always rises. That my worth is more than we can ever imagine. And even when we make mistakes or doubt ourselves that you are there to remind us just how worthy we are.

Affirmation to speaking life:

I am stronger than any storms

Song to add to playlist: The Sun is Rising - Britt Nicole

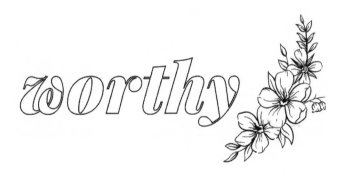

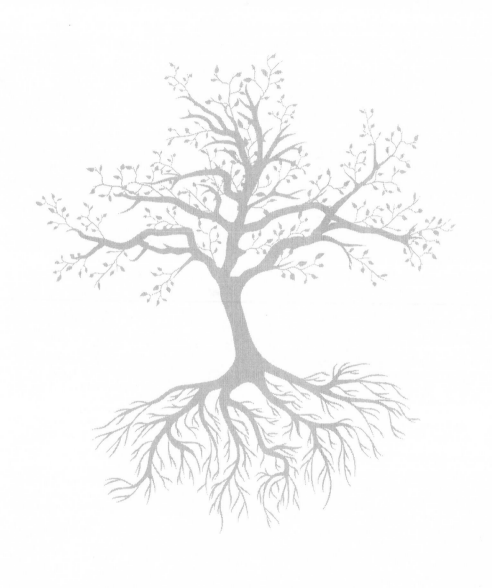

Rare Jewels

Day 5

The stone the builders rejected has become the cornerstone; the Lord has
done this and it is marvelous in our eyes.

- Matthew 21:42

These days, social media has become where you find your identity, value and
comparison. We measure our worth with what people say about us. And we allow
trends, likes and comments to fulfill us. For we do not want to be rejected, but often
social media is just filtered lies.

In 1996, I was diagnosed with anorexia nervosa. I was only 14 years old. But, at
14, the trend was to be super skinny. I had been a soccer player since the age of 3. I
was curvy and my quads were huge. My worth and identity was caught up in being
skinny. I felt like an outcast. So, to fit in and not be rejected, I started to control what
would allow me to be skinny. That was food. But, what I didn't know and what
I tell all my young ladies is you were created to stand out. If someone rejects or
doesn't accept you it's ok. You were made so special and so unique, that often times
you forget that. We allow others, and sometimes ourselves, to say things that aren't
even true. And it will be remembered in a few years, if you give it power. But, take
a minute to speak life and truly look, you will see even if you feel rejected, that you
are God's cornerstone, a marvelous masterpiece. It took me 7 years to beat my eating
disorder and learn that what I may say isn't what God says.

QUESTION: What is something you are comparing yourself to?

_____

_____

_____

_____

_____

_____

_____

_____

_____

_____

_____

_____

_____

_____

_____

_____

_____

_____

_____

_____

_____

_____

_____

_____

PRAYER: Father, I ask that you remove any lie that has been spoken over me. I ask that you remind me each day of how I am yours. That when social media creeps in, you redirect my thoughts to who I truly am. A precious jewel created by you. Thank you for saying I am yours. Amen

Affirmation to speaking life:

I am not what was spoken over me.

Song to add to playlist: You Say - Lauren Daigle

Mindfulness pose: Tree pose you are strong and rooted hold for 10 breaths repeat for 3

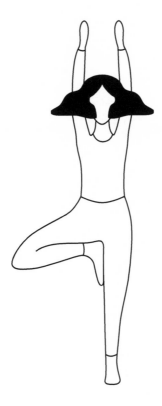

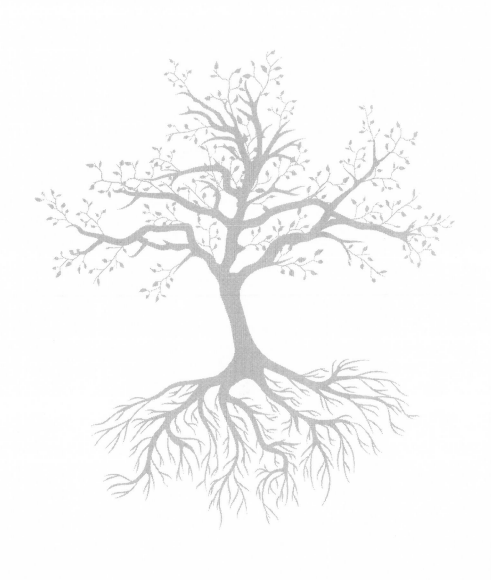

Holding onto the Life Raft

Day 6:

Even though you slay me, I will trust in him.

- Job 13

Ever feel like you are just drowning? That every time you get back up more comes at you? So much darkness and you can't find the light at the end of the tunnel? As I write this, I will share that this is where I am right now. Every day it's another arrow, another blow. But even through all of this I am reminded of all the other times He has brought me through and has helped me to rise. Every valley you walk through, you are never truly alone and even when you struggle, hope and trust in Him will bring you through.

QUESTION: Can you release whatever you are going through to Him?

_____

_____

_____

_____

_____

_____

_____

_____

_____

_____

_____

_____

_____

_____

_____

_____

_____

_____

_____

_____

_____

_____

PRAYER: Lord, for you know what I am going through. Even though you know the outcome I ask that you speak life into me so that I may keep going. That even though I feel my world is imploding that you help me trust in you and give me hope that this is just a season.

Affirmation to speaking life:

I will trust, walk in faith, and believe in His promises.

Song to add to playlist: Another in the Fire - Hillsong

Quote: You will not fear the terror of night, nor the arrow that flies by day.

- Psalms 91:5

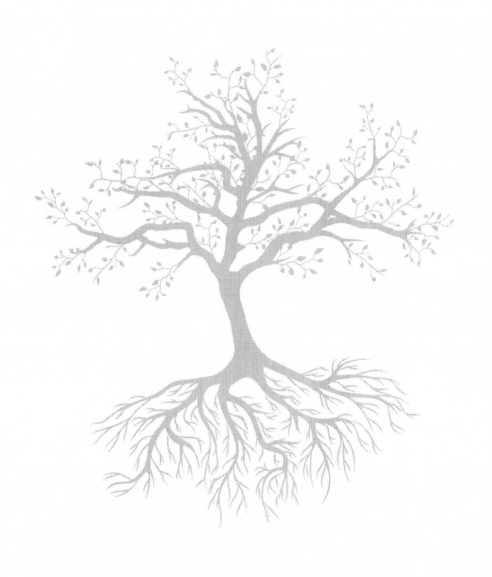

All the Desires

Day 7

Delight yourself in the Lord and He will give you the desires of your heart.
- Psalms 37:4

"Desires of the heart." At 13 I read that verse as I was popping my bubblicious gum doing my homework of memorizing this bible verse. I thought this is like getting everything I have ever wanted. All the while, staring at my JTT poster dreaming of one day making it to hollywood.

So, I sang my little heart out at church that Sunday, watched the kids in Sunday school and later that night I was going to pray for my greatest desire - That my crush, I had at 13, would be my boyfriend. That is what that verse said, right? If I praise and do good things, God will grant me anything my heart desires.

How many times have we gone to God asking him for things, like a kid does when he goes and sees Santa to tell him what he wants for cChristmas?

But, if you truly read Psalms 37, you will see the words, to trust, to commit, to delight, to be still, but most importantly, to be patient. See, Ie skipped all those words and went straight to, "Hey God, it's me again. So that boy I like, ummm, when will he be my boyfriend? I did what you said." But, do we truly delight in Him during the hard times, the uncontrollable seasons, the times where all you can do is say, "Lord, hey, I need just you." Or do you get that prayer answered and say, "Yo, God, I see you. Go ahead, I will catch you next time when I need something answered."

I never got that crush to be my boyfriend and I was upset with God for not granting my desire and for getting my feelings hurt. As I sat at Burger King with my dad, crying my eyes out, drinking a strawberry milkshake, I learned a valuable lesson: My worth and value didnt come from others, and God isn't a genie who grants wishes.

QUESTION: What is something you have prayed about but God hasn't answered? Is it something you desire that is beneficial to giving you joy? Is it something you have a string attached saying, "if you answer, I promise to serve you?" _____

_____

_____

_____

_____

_____

_____

_____

_____

_____

_____

_____

_____

_____

_____

_____

_____

_____

_____

_____

_____

_____

_____

_____

PRAYER: Lord, for you know the desires of my heart. You know what Ie need before I even ask it. I ask you, Lord to help me to truly delight in you, to learn to let go and trust that you know what will work for me, but also to have patience as I wait for you to answer

Affirmation to speaking life:

I put my trust in God

Song to add to playlist: Glorify - Jordan Feliz

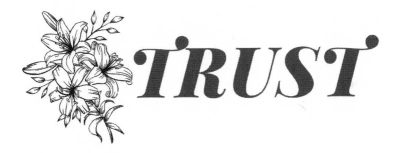

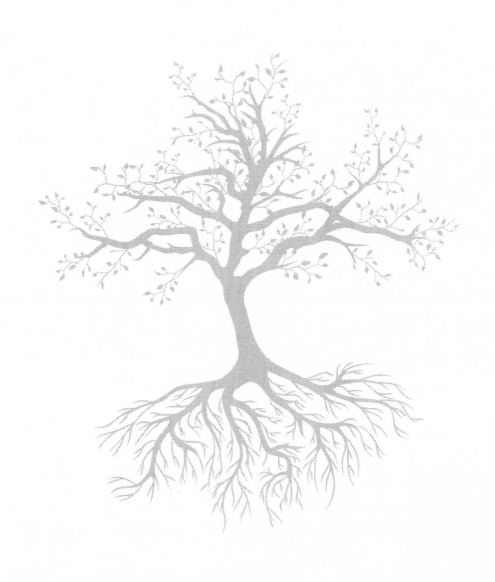

Trying to Understand

Day 8

Trust in the Lord with all your heart and lean not on your own understanding;
in all your ways submit, to him and he will make your paths straight - Proverbs 3:5-6

Trust is the one word that we hold so close to our heart and give so freely. How many times have you said, "Oh girl, you know I trust you, or you can trust me"? and when we were upset or felt betrayed, you broke my trust.

Trust is something I truly struggle with. Through all of the heart breaks, set backs, and lessons, every time, I try to figure out and understand. I had God speaking, "Do you trust me?"

During March 2020, the world shutdown and I sat in my gym telling the last member that we would be shutting down. I sat on that turf with tears running down my face saying, "God now what do I do? We won't make it. We have only been open for a short time." As I sat in my gym pleading and trying to make a way out of the unknown. I heard him say, "Trust me, Paola."

The shutdown taught me one thing as a small business owner. That trust and faith are the true currency that brought us through. Everytime I tried to understand, I would get defeated and upset. Trust me, letting go isn't easy. Fully trusting and saying, "Hey there, God, here you go, we had to freeze all memberships. Welp, how do we pay these bills?" And something amazing happened, He always made a way.

Rise was one of the fortunate businesses that got to open its doors back up. Everytime I think of that moment on the turf, I sit back in wonder. Even though I can't grasp it, I do know trust and walking in faith.

SO, today the question is how is it we give our trust so freely, yet when it comes to truly trusting in our Waymaker, we struggle to release that trust? _____

_____

_____

_____

_____

_____

_____

_____

_____

_____

_____

_____

_____

_____

_____

_____

_____

_____

_____

_____

_____

_____

_____

_____

PRAYER: Lord, I ask you to help me to not lean on my own understanding, but to be able to trust you so freely like I trust others so easily. That whatever I am battling or going through, I release control and allow you to amaze me.

Affirmation to speaking life:

I release the things I do not understand and choose to walk in faith.

Song to add to playlist: Waymaker - Leeland

Mindfulness pose: Downward dog hold for 10 breaths release repeat for 3

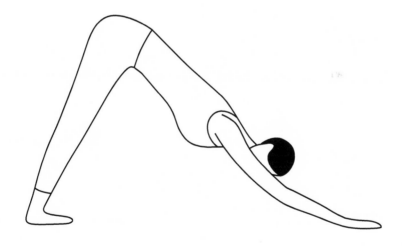

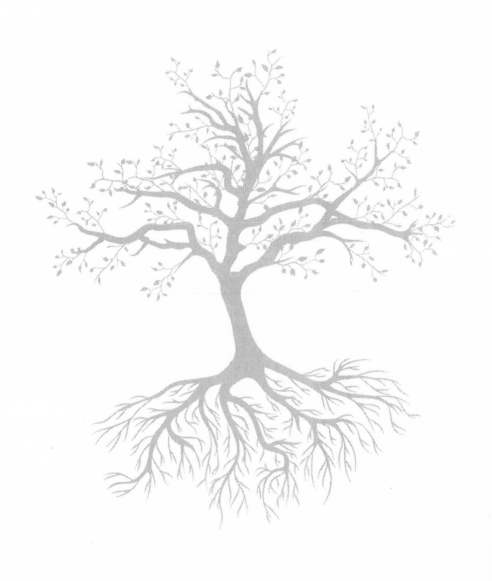

Oops, I did it Again

Day 9

Cast all your anxiety on Him because He cares for you.

- 1 Peter 5:7

"Hey God, Knock knock."

God: "Hi, Paola"

Me: "Welp, you know it's me again God. You know I did it again. So I guess I should just let You take over now."

God: "So, now you are ready to trust in me again?"

Me (sheepishly smiles), "Yea, I tried, but you know I should of just handed it over."

That's how I imagine it goes everytime I stumble and fall. I get up and try again and fail some more. Then, when I am finally ready to say,"Jesus, please take the wheel", my knock knock jokes with God starts.

I mean, I know I'm not the only one that feels like a little kid going to see their parents about something they know you are hiding and try to crack a joke. I'm glad God loves my knock knock jokes. But, seriously, how amazing is it that even though we screw up and we try to take control, God is always there. Ready to take over and give us the peace that everything will be ok. No matter the situation, He is there like, "I got you, I got this. Go rest girl."

QUESTION: What are you currently trying to handle, that you know God should be handling? What knock knock joke would you do ask you hand over your problems to God?

_____

_____

_____

_____

_____

_____

_____

_____

_____

_____

_____

_____

_____

_____

_____

_____

_____

_____

_____

_____

_____

_____

_____

PRAYER: God, your words say to cast all my cares upon you. Sometimes I am so quick to cast all of my cares. But, sometimes, I am so ashamed of some of the situations I created so instead of letting You help, I hold onto those burdens. Lord, I ask that you help me to surrender all burdens to you. That, as I struggle to release the control, you are there reminding me that you are here for me and not against me. I just thank you for giving me grace and understanding, but most importantly, that you love me: flaws and all. In Jesus name I pray, amen.

Affirmation to speaking life:

It's ok to not have it all together, but I am enough

Song to add to playlist: Overcomer - Mandisa

Quote: Do not worry about tomorrow, for tomorrow is always brand new.

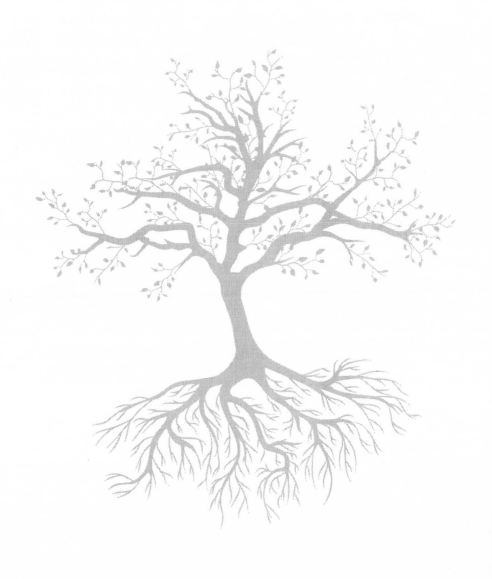

Testing Faith

Day 10

"Have faith in God," Jesus answered. "Truly I tell you, if anyone says to this
mountain, 'Go, throw yourself into the sea,' and does not doubt in their heart,
but believes that what they say will happen, it will be done for them.
Therefore I tell you, whatever you ask for in prayer, believe that you
have received it, and it will be yours.

Mark 11: 22 - 24

We get so caught up on the things we don't have. Of the prayers that haven't been
answered. That we don't take a moment to see all the things that have been answered.
We forget to see the miracles, the restorations, the healing and the opportunities he
has done for us. So, if he has answered before my friend, don't you know that with
the same faith, he will answer again?

So do not waiver, do not get upset or stressed because if you believe it, it will be
answered. Just remember, sometimes it's not the answer you might want. Sometimes,
it's an answer that you never thought possible. So, let's count and enjoy all those
blessings and walk in that faith!

QUESTION: What is an answered prayer that left you in awe? Can you take a walk through that answered prayer and list the blessings that came out of it?

_____

_____

_____

_____

_____

_____

_____

_____

_____

_____

_____

_____

_____

_____

_____

_____

_____

_____

_____

_____

_____

_____

_____

PRAYER: Lord, thank you for everything you have done for me. For every prayer answered, that even when I wavered and doubted you, still came through. I thank you and praise you for the future prayers. Thank you for closing doors that I didn't know that needed to be closed, but opened new ones that I never thought about. Amen

Affirmation to Speaking life :

I am blessed beyond all measure

Song to add to playlist: Counting Every Blessing - Rend Collective

Mindfulness pose: Forward fold (or half fold) hold for 10 sec release repeat for 3

You did not choose me, but I choose you and appointed so that you might go and bear fruit - fruit that will last. - John 15:16

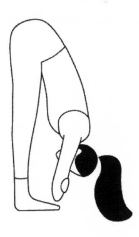

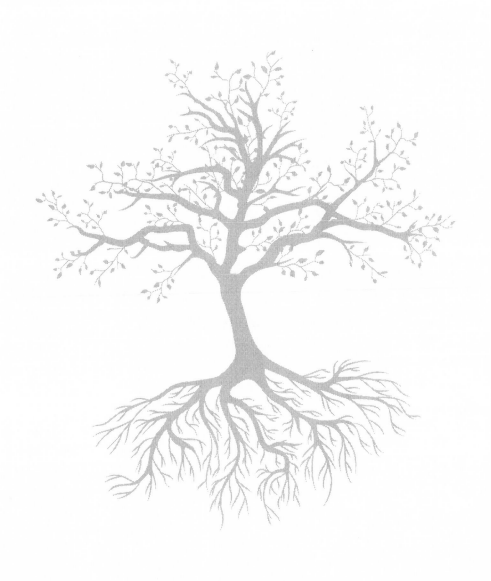

These next few days are some deep ones. I had to pray about sharing some of this but when God says, "it's time", well here I am, sharing some parts of me. So here we go:

Days 12-18 are a look into how my faith was shaped and developed from one tragic loss to taking that big risk and always wondering. Even with how broken I am, can He truly use me, to learning to trust Him through all of my storms, and planting little mustard seeds. These are days that I come back to during the quiet moments, where I reflect am I doing enough of shining His light. No matter what God has in store for you, remember no matter how great the loss, you are always able to take what you have been through and share. All it takes in this world, is helping one person to shine their beautiful light .

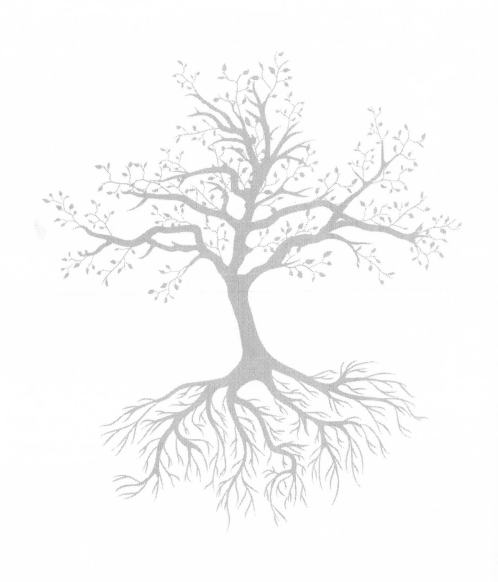

Risk Taker

Day 11:

I can do all things through Christ that gives me strength.

- Philippians 4:13

How many times have we said...."oh I can't do that?" I wish, but I am too old, not strong enough or I dont have the skills or talent to do that. Why do we speak so much negativity? We know that if we just try, we might surprise ourselves?

Many know that I am a risk taker. I am not a planner. I live my life just winging it. I know this little, but awesome, piece of me drives my husband nuts. He is the planner and I'm always at the last random minute. "Hey, let's go do this."

Maybe it's the days in Sunday school where I heard this verse. And as I was learning to ride my bike, at the fun age of 5, my dad was holding on the bike saying, "Paola, you can do it." I remember looking back screaming, "I can do all things through Christ!" And went head first into the bus stop! I still laugh at my 5 year old self, no fear, just excitement to take the training wheels off. But, I know this is the moment where the risk taker was bloomed and rooted.

So, why can't you let that inner child, that had all that wonder and excitement, and no fear, try something? What's the worst that can happen if you fail? Guess what, you may fail, like I did with that bus stop. But, just like I did , you tried and that's the best feeling!

QUESTION: What is something you always wanted to do, but you keep holding yourself back? _____

_____

_____

_____

_____

_____

_____

_____

_____

_____

_____

_____

_____

_____

_____

_____

_____

_____

_____

_____

_____

_____

_____

_____

PRAYER: Thank you Lord for reminding me how, with you and the right mindset, I can do all things. Remove all negativity that gives me fear and doubt. For that doesnt come from you. For you give us strength and purpose. In Jesus name, Amen.

Affirmation to speaking life:

You can do all things

Song to add to playlist: Get Back Up - TobyMac

Drawing to color

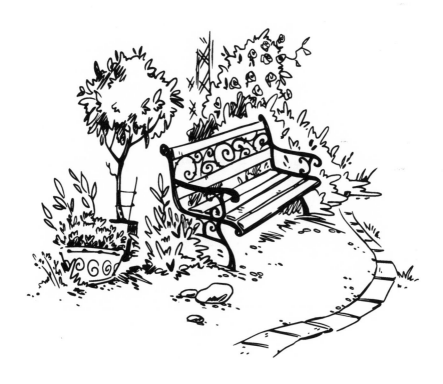

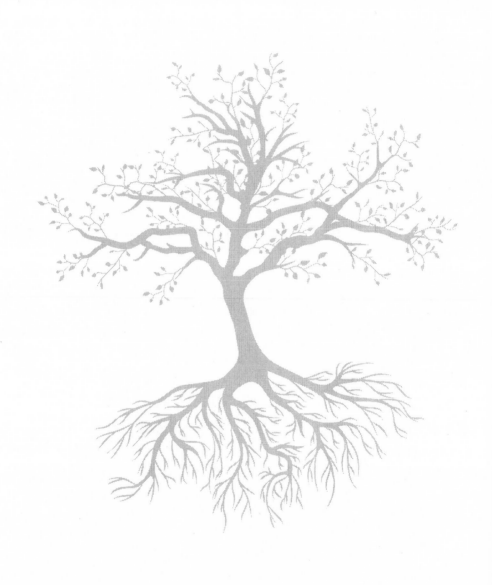

Thy Will

Day 12

For the righteous fall seven times, they rise again.

\- Proverbs 24:16

I can count on my hands how many times I have felt like my world was destroyed and that my life was over. Like, this 12th day is a hard one. This is where I was ready for God to just take me and this day back.

Every year, since December 12, 2017, I have struggled. I struggle with failure, with heartache and emptiness. On that day I lost my son. It was so unexpected. But, to this day I can still feel and hear that scream and watch my husband run into the bathroom. I remember in slow motion seeing this tiny little person, with his tiny little hands and I remember staring at his hands knowing that he will never hold my hand back.

But, what no one truly knows is how bad I had fallen. I remember sitting on the bathroom floor with a bottle of Oxy that they had sent me home with, feeling so numb. I sat there opening that bottle and pouring that whole bottle into my hand and calling God a liar as I screamed Jeremiah 29:11 was nothing but a lie. I sat there rocking, saying, "Just take me, if that is truly what you want, just take me." I battled losing time as I played with those pills telling God how I shouldn't be shocked that He took his own son, so why wouldn't he take mine.

As I laid on that floor in tears, that first pill kicked in, and I slipped into a quiet sleep. As I slept, I found myself on a bridge, but I couldn't move. As I looked at the field in front of me, I saw a black labrador running in the field, chasing a curly-haired toddler that was laughing and giggling. The dog ran to that bridge and as I pet him I realized that the dog was KC, our family dog. As he ran back to the field, I tried to chase him, because I knew in my heart that the little boy was Kellen. As I tried to run over that bridge, I was pushed back. I screamed for God to let me pass and Jesus crossed over to me and said, "Your son Kellen is ok, but my purpose for you isn't finished." I started to beg and cry. Begging to let me stay with him. Kellen turned with the sweetest smile and waved. Jesus said, "Paola, my plans and purpose for you aren't over. Kellen is where he needs to be." And as they walked away Jesus gently said, "It's time for you to rise."

I woke up with those pills in my hands and flushed them down the toilet. A few days later, on Christmas eve, Damian handed me over a binder that had a business plan and 3 little stocks the name of the business Rise Above the Ashes Fitness.

I share this with you, my friends, as a simple reminder. You may feel like everything is over, that there is nothing to live for anymore. But, I am here testifying to you that you will make it through. It is not easy, I still struggle, but with faith you will make it.

QUESTION: Look back at a dark time. Can you remember how you made it through?

_____

_____

_____

_____

_____

_____

_____

_____

_____

_____

_____

_____

_____

_____

_____

PRAYER: Lord, we do not understand why things happen the way they do. But, we know that you will see us through. That even when we are ready to give up you will make a way for us to keep going. Whatever my friends are going through, help them to trust in you, Amen

Song to add to playlist: Thy Will - Hillary Scott

Affirmation to speaking life:

I will get through this and Rise

Mindfulness pose: Butterfly pose hold for 10 secs repeat for 3 sets

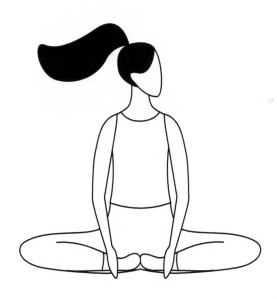

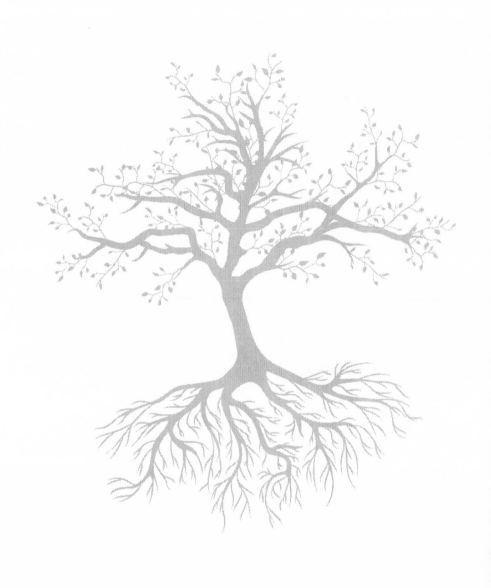

Even if We are Thrown into the Blazing Fire

Day 13

If we are thrown into the blazing furnace, the God we serve is able to deliver us
from it, and He will deliver us from Your Majesty's hand. But even if He does not,
we want you to know. - Daniel 3:17-18

It makes no sense why God does the things He does, right? I mean, that is what we try to tell ourselves. But, after the loss of my son Kellen, I found myself asking God what was the reason and why He didn't just take me. As everyone knows from day 12, Rise was born.

There will always be moments in our lives where we will question or want to give up. But even if that is how you are feeling, know that the true test of faith is during the storms in our lives. I catch myself during moments in times I don't understand, I want to waive that surrender flag. Even at my worst, if this is part of the plan I will still trust and walk with faith. Because, if I had given up, I know that Rise wouldn't be here making the impact that it does.

Growing up, looking back, I thought something we often all do. When life is great, why don't we take the time to pray and praise Him. Almost losing my marriage in 2009 and losing my son in 2017 has taught me it doesn't matter if your life is hard, easy, blessed beyond measure, you continue to pray, trust and believe. Just like Shadrach, Meshach, and Abednego were thrown into that furnace, they knew He never left them, they trusted and continued to praise Him.

QUESTION: What is one thing you are struggling with and questioning God about? Can you release it and truly trust Him during that hard walk in the fire?

_____

_____

_____

_____

_____

_____

_____

_____

_____

_____

_____

_____

_____

_____

_____

_____

_____

_____

_____

_____

_____

_____

_____

PRAYER: Lord help me to not ask why, but to be able to pray and still walk in faith. Even if I struggle with the outcomes I will still continue to trust in you! Amen

Affirmation to speaking life:

Even if I struggle, I know You have me during all my seasons and like a phoenix, I will rise from the ashes.

Song to add to playlist: Even If - Mercy Me

Quote: For everyone rises through the ashes, for He makes beauty from those same ashes….so smile and rise. - Paola

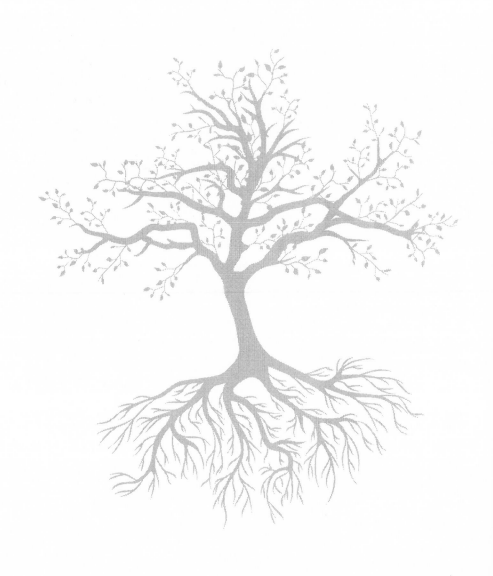

Planting Mustard Seeds

Day 14

If you have faith as small as a mustard seed, you can tell this mountain to move from here to there, and it moves. Nothing will be impossible for you.

- Matthew 17:20-21

Oh, how I love this verse. Faith as small as a mustard seed. My whole life every little thing that I thought could never happen or possible I have seen it bloom and blossom. As I sit here writing this daily journal, I smile with tears and wonder. Because, God used this broken, hot mess, never perfect girl like me to shine His light. And when I had such little faith, He always reminded me it was enough faith to water that mustard seed.

So, my friend, if you think you are too broken to ever be used, know that He can and will use you. Your brokenness is part of your story and is meant to make that mustard seed bloom into something more than you can ever imagine.

QUESTION: What is something you are trusting God to answer? Are you trusting no matter how much faith you have? _____

_____

_____

_____

_____

_____

_____

_____

_____

_____

_____

_____

_____

_____

_____

_____

_____

_____

_____

_____

_____

_____

_____

_____

PRAYER: Lord no matter how small faith I may have, remind me of all the little seedlings you have planted for me. Thank you for always giving me hope in all things. Even when I struggle I know you are there helping me tend my garden.

Affirmation to speaking life:

No matter how broken I am, I am able to plant a beautiful story with my mustard seed of faith.

Song to add to playlist: My Jesus - Anne Wilson

Drawing: little seedlings of mustard seeds

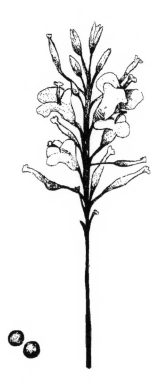

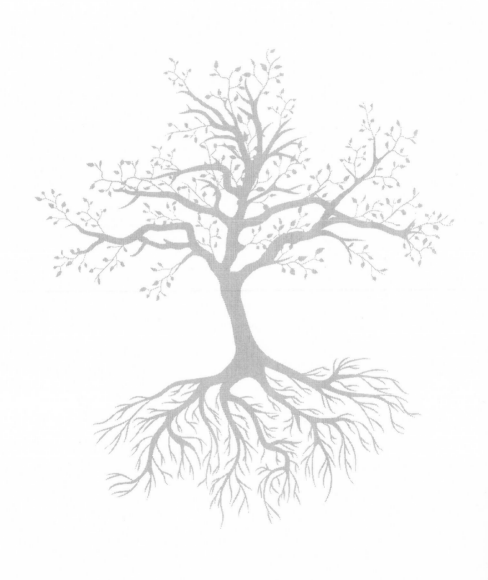

Shine Your Light

Day 15

Let your light shine before others, that they may see your good deeds
and glorify your Father in heaven.

- Matthew 5:16

We ALL have such a beautiful light inside of us. A light meant to help light others and shine for His glory. But, I am so guilty for letting my light hide. For a long time, I allowed my fear of what others thought or the things I have been through, to stop me from shining that light of mine.

To this day, I love to be behind the scenes at Rise. And on my own platforms. Even now, as I write this, I have an anxiety of being mocked or ridiculed. It's pretty silly right?

But for a majority of us, we allow social media, friends, family and people we truly do not know.stop us from doing things, sharing our stories or even stepping out of comfort zones.

In Sunday school, I would pray to not be called on to read the Bible verse. But, when it was time to sing this little light of mine, I would sing like I was about to audition for American Idol! I may have been off key, but when it got to, "Don't let Satan blow it out, I'm going to let it shine." I belted that verse like I had won a prize.

So why do we allow all these doubts, opinions hinder us? Your little light was meant to light others and make a ripple of lights shining all around you? As I write this, I'm over here saying, "it's time to keep letting your light shine." My friends, you were meant to rise and shine and do such great things.

QUESTION: Aare you allowing what others will think dim your light?

_____

_____

_____

_____

_____

_____

_____

_____

_____

_____

_____

_____

_____

_____

_____

_____

_____

_____

_____

_____

_____

_____

_____

_____

_____

PRAYER: Lord help me to shine my little light. When I want to shrink or hide my light, remind me that nothing should hinder doing your purpose for me.

Affirmations to speaking life:

For I am a rare light meant to shine and light the world

Song to add to playlist: Stars go Dim - Better

Mindfulness pose: warrior 1 hold for 10 seconds 3 repetitions each side

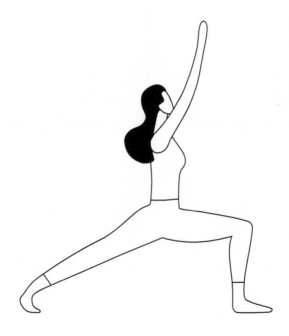

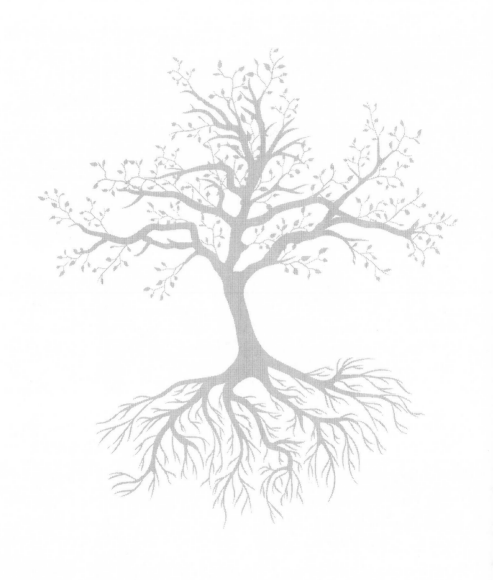

What Do I Have to Offer?

Day 16

Here is a boy with five small barley loaves and two small fish, but how
far will they go among so many? - John 6:9

You have these great ideas, dreams and aspirations. But, everything costs money and everything takes a risk. Will it succeed or fail? Then, you find yourself asking, "well how can I truly be used to serving when I truly lack the funds?"

I have been that person, and said those exact things. But, probably more jokingly, like, "God excuse me? You want me to do what? Repeat that for me one more time. You want me to open my first hub, a gym in a town that I know nobody? You want me to leap from this comfortable job and chase this passion? And how do you want me to do this exactly," as I laugh and shake my head at God.

Because God says to me, "Oh ye of little faith, it has already been planned." The question is do you believe and have the faith that it is possible? And are you willing to step out in faith away from that comfort zone and do it?

The joke is on me, huh? Because, my friend, Rise is my 5 loaves of barley and two fishes. The day my husband handed me over that business plan with a check from his 401k and the little check left from my 401k,. I looked at my husband like he was crazy! But, from the space that it started to the current space, everytime I see it, I walk in and I'm reminded of this Bible verse. Because, even when we had no funds, God came through and made it happen.

There was a moment when I was given the opportunity to move up to its current location. I went through the process of adding an investor or taking a loan because that space would need more equipment. And with every door that closed in my face, I was getting so frustrated. And God said, "So, when will you stop relying on men, when I have carried you this far." 5 loaves and 2 fishes! Even today as we went through a shutdown, freezing memberships, losing members, denial to all bailouts. We opened back up and thought we were just making it. I give thanks for His promises He has for me and for my 5 loaves and 2 fishes.

I share this because, I have waivered. I have had my doubts on everything. I have sat on my turf in tears wondering how I was going to pay a bill or how this gym was going to make it. Not because I was afraid of losing it, but, because of the people who have found a refuge in Rise. How God was able to use this broken girl with His 5 loaves and 2 fishes to shine His light.

So my friends take that risk. God has mighty plans for your 5 loaves and 2 fishes to shine His light and to make an impact no matter how small or big. It will eventually set a fire to touch a multitude.

QUESTION: Do you have a purpose that you want to share, but aren't sure how you can use it? _____

_____

_____

_____

_____

_____

_____

_____

_____

_____

_____

_____

_____

PRAYER: Lord, thank you for reminding us how you can use us, and how you can provide for us. Our purpose and dreams, when guided by you, will flourish more than we could ever imagine. Even when we see it impossible, you make it possible. Amen

Affirmation to speaking life:

I am possible
My purpose is possible

Song to add to playlist: Look What You've Done - Tasha Layton

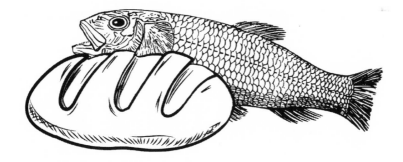

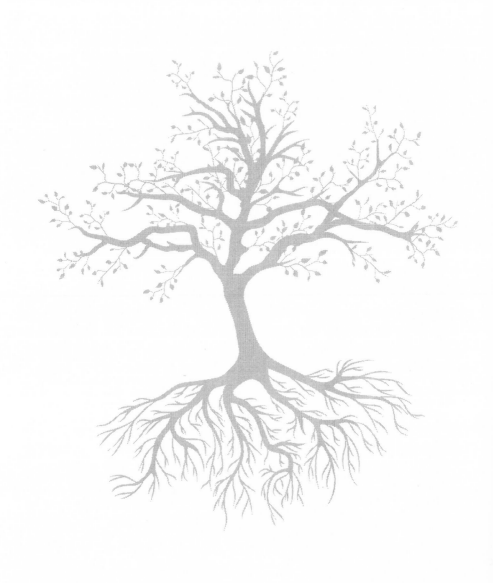

Will He Still Use Me?

Day 17

Come see a man who told me everything, I ever did.

- John 4:29

We hear the stories of some amazing women in the Bible, like Ruth, Esther, and Sarah. We often find ourselves saying, "I want to be that Proverbs 31 woman." How God used them despite everything going on is remarkable to me. But, the one woman that is in the Bible that I truly love is the Samaritan Woman, at the well ,who met "Jesus. He told me everything I did!" She exclaimed in awe. She wondered if she was truly speaking to the King of Kings, the Messiah.

Never once judging her for her past or present, and giving nothing but grace, mercy and waiting for her to let Him be part of her future. Even as his disciples came back, they never once said, "hey why are you talking to her?" Or "Hey lady, why are you bugging him? He hasn't eaten. They stood by his side listening to him, as he treated her with such grace, not judging, not looking at her, because she was a Samaritan.

So, I find myself wondering why we are so quick to judge one another for every wrong doing and give no mercy or grace? But, also why do we allow what has happened to us in our past to not extend grace upon ourselves?

My friends, that woman at the well, are all of us. It doesn't matter how broken, how messed up , how much wrong doing you have done, and the screwups we fester on. Jesus can still use you. Just like He did with her to spread his love, mercy and grace.

Believe me, for I have been that woman. I am still her. And everytime I stumble or go my own way, God is still there, meeting me at the well and pouring so much grace and mercy into me. And it's so amazing.

QUESTION: Can you let go of that one root that is holding you back from believing you can still be used? _____

_____

_____

_____

_____

_____

_____

_____

_____

_____

_____

_____

_____

_____

_____

_____

_____

_____

_____

_____

_____

_____

_____

_____

_____

Affirmation to speaking life:

No matter how broken, I can be used for His glory

Song to add to playlist: Women at the Well - Olivia Lane

Mindfulness pose: child pose - Hold for 10 breaths repeat for 3

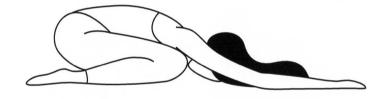

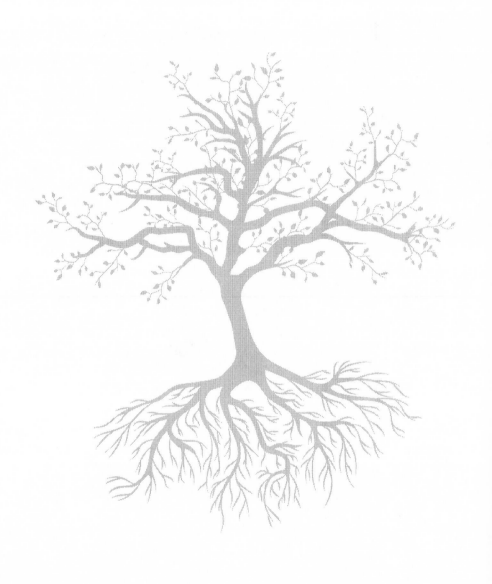

Restored

Day 18

And the God of grace who called you to His eternal glory in Christ, after you suffered
a little while., will himself restore you, and make you strong, firm steadfast. - 1 Peter 5:10

Whoa! Take a moment to read that verse again! When I read this I got chills.
Because man, has God restored, redeemed and made this girl stronger than she could
ever imagine. My story is one I always ask, "God how am I still here standing?" I
used to have so much shame with some of the things I have been through, but I know
God has me sharing this because there is someone out there that has either gone
through it, or is going through it and feels so alone and ready to give up. Don't give
up because you're not alone in love. And even though this is hard for me to share
with my friends, this is why I love how God gives me so much strength and grace.

God took a girl who was sexually assaulted at the age of 4, to being diagnosed
with anorexia nervosa at the age of 14, from a teen mom at the age of 18. That same
son was diagnosed with aspergers at 23. To watch her marriage crumble and lead to
divorce at 26. To help her heal from her body dysmorphia and find herself and give
her a purpose at 26. To go through a possible ovarian cancer scare at 26, that later led
to the loss of a son at 33. To opening a gym, in his memory and watching it struggle,
and going through my own growing pains, and watching the lights go out, as she
closes her door through a pandemic. And now, I am in a new season in year 38, as I
write this during another hard storm and season. I look back at each moment, each
season, each moment of fear I had and smile. Because, when I thought each season
was my downfall and I will never survive. He brought me through it and I can't
praise or thank him enough.

My sweet friends, know that your story and seasons will always be what makes
you you. But, being redeemed, restored and being able to use your story to help

others is the true strength of God. Restoring you, healing you because, He loves you and never forgot about you. He was the one carrying you through all the past, present and future seasons.

QUESTION: Looking back during the suffering and storms, do you now see how valuable and precious you are? That He will restore you?

_____

_____

_____

_____

_____

_____

_____

_____

_____

_____

_____

_____

_____

_____

_____

_____

_____

_____

_____

_____

Affirmation to speaking life:

I am redeemed

Songs to add to playlist: Great Are You Lord & Rescue - Lauren Daigle

Quote: No matter how broken you feel or the flaws that you are ashamed of. These things are what makes your restoration so beautiful and unique - Paola Leimenstoll

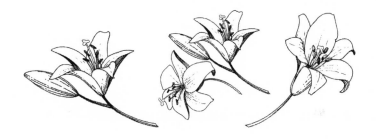

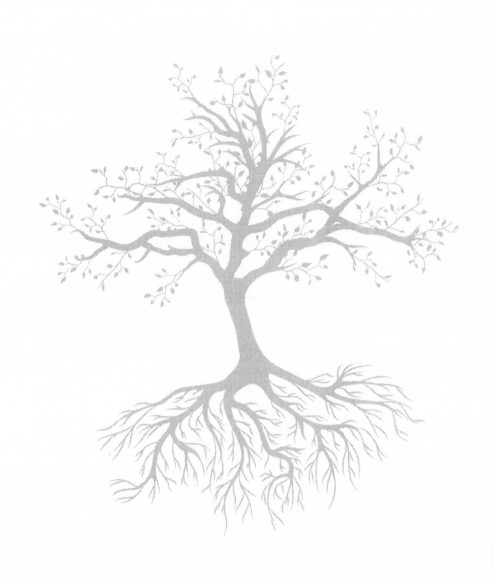

The part of the healing that is the most uncomfortable, but it is part of helping you be able to help shine your light. Forgiveness, judging, boundaries these are some of the things I struggle with. But, it's ok to not be perfect, just take a moment to pray, release and let God. Because, let's be real, if I was perfect, well what use will God have for me? Just part of the flaws of raising my friends.

Welcome to days 19-21…deep breaths!

Not that I have already obtained this or am perfect, but I press on to make it my own. Because Christ Jesus has made me His own. But, one thing I do: forgetting what lies behind and straining forward to what lies ahead, I press on towards the goal for the prize of the upward call of God in Christ Jesus. Let those of us who are mature think this way, and if anything you think otherwise, God will reveal that also to you.

Philippians 3:12-13

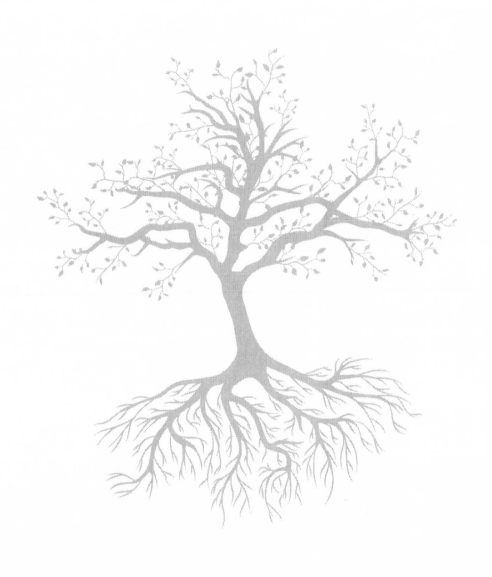

Forgiveness

Day19

Get rid of all bitterness, rage and anger, brawling slander along with every form
of malice be kind and compassionate to one another, forgiving each other, just as Christ
has forgave you. - Ephesians 4:31-32

Welp, let me start by saying that,"Boy, do I screw that verse up! I mean, when God
says to turn the cheek and to forgive 7x77, lets just say, I turn into Sophia from Golden
Girls. I have a memory lapse while letting that Latin temper and tongue lashing come
out. I did say I wasn't perfect and I do get, "Wait, I thought you were a Christian?"
Well yes, I am, but I make mistakes along the way.

There are daily conversations that I have with God. Even reminding Him that
when He decided to create me, He made me Latin! Then God reminds me of allowing
mercy and grace. So then I say, "I can forgive and forget and pray, but can I just check
them?" And then here comes God checking ME and putting me in time out saying,
"So would you like me to check you?"

"Oh, ok God, we are going *that* direction?" Well ,let me just go over here and mop
this floor with bleach and Fabuloso and just pray. Because, today isn't the day I want
to be checked by you ,Lord. I'm just going to start dishing out all the forgiveness.

I know my friends, I'm not the only one having these conversations. There are days
I just say, "Lord can't I just be a tiny bit hood and a lot of holy?" If God gave eyerolls
I know I would have a ton of those in my direction! lol. And He says, "Paola, forgive,
turn your cheek and let's move on."

So, today I challenge you instead of that Sophia quick-tongue, speak life into that
situation. Forgive so you can move on. The best prayers are done while cleaning and
using that Fabuloso and bleach. I mean, because the best thing when you forgive,
is not just releasing them from anything you did, but it is also releasing you from
anything you may have done, as well. Oh, trust me, that was hard to write. I know I

am stubborn and caused some of it, that probably took me a lot of Fabulosos to come to admitting that. So, put the hoop earrings up, take a deep breath and smell the Fabuloso. Also a great, "I'm sorry, please forgive me," is a few bottles of Fabuloso. Everyone loves the smell of cleanliness and you are cleaning out the unforgiveness to let God use you just a little bit more.

QUESTION: Are you busy holding onto something that was done to you? Instead of talking to God about it to help you to release and let go? How about you struggling to forgive yourself for something you put yourself through?

_____

_____

_____

_____

_____

_____

_____

_____

_____

_____

_____

_____

_____

_____

_____

_____

_____

_____

PRAYER: Lord, help me to forgive when I do not want to forgive. Help me to be able to take a deep breath and turn that cheek, even when those hoop earrings want to come off. In Jesus name, amen

Affirmation to speaking life:

To forgive clears my soul

Song to add to playlist: O Come to the Altar - Elevation Worship

Mindfulness pose: Shavasana

Lie with your eyes close for 1 minute think of what needs to be let go take a deep breath and exhale that release as you inhale think of something that will bring you joy.

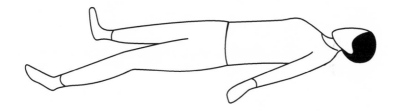

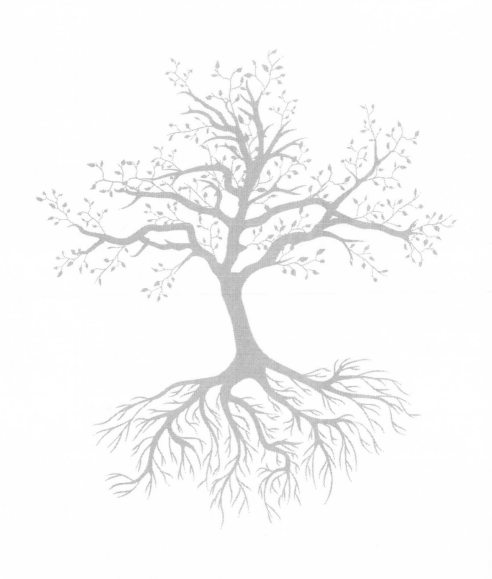

Oh No, She Didnt

Day 20

Do not judge or you will be judged. For the same way you judge others you
will be judged. And with the measure you use it , will be measured to you. - Matthew 7:1-2

One, this is one hard pill to swallow. It is so easy to look back and see the times I have been caught up on the judgment train. Where someone points someone out and you listen to all the things they have to say. Or you listen to the hearsay they heard about you. And sometimes you are the one venting out the frustrations of pettiness.

Growing up, my parents always told us to not focus on what others say or do to us. One thing that has stuck to me when you point the finger or point something out is how many of those fingers are being pointed back at you?

I try this, but instead I'm hard headed and it takes me a few tries. I think I took my other lesson that my dad told me to never take no crap from nobody and used that a little bit more. But, as I have gotten older, I have grown tired with how easy it is to get into cliques, or to join in with the ones who decide to not like someone. Sadly, I have been on both sides and it isn't fun. The things I have heard about me, have many times had me question why I do what I do.

The truth I have come to learn is quite simple. We honestly don't know what a person is going through. We do not know their storms or what burdens they are carrying. We are all human and we truly make mistakes. Believe me, God knows and has reminded me of the times I wasn't my best.

Judging is so easy to do with social media, screen shots, rumors and gossip. But, we all need to truly remind ourselves that before we point and cast that stone is our home free of clutter and perfect? If we were truly perfect, we would be like Jesus, right? So let's start breaking those chains of judging others and start speaking life and throwing kindness around. The world needs that more than ever.

QUESTION: Before you speak or join in or even hear what has been said about you, will it build you or that person up? _____

_____

_____

_____

_____

_____

_____

_____

_____

_____

_____

_____

_____

_____

_____

_____

_____

_____

_____

_____

_____

_____

_____

_____

PRAYER: Lord, help me to do better when it comes to others. When we know how easy it is to fall into judging and gossiping, it helps us to pause and speak life into the conversation instead of slander. In Jesus name, amen

Affirmation to speaking life:

I will choose to speak life

Song to add to playlist: Not Backing Down - Blanca

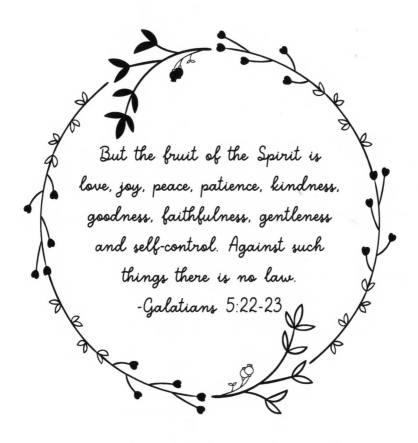

But the fruit of the Spirit is
love, joy, peace, patience, kindness,
goodness, faithfulness, gentleness
and self-control. Against such
things there is no law.
-Galatians 5:22-23

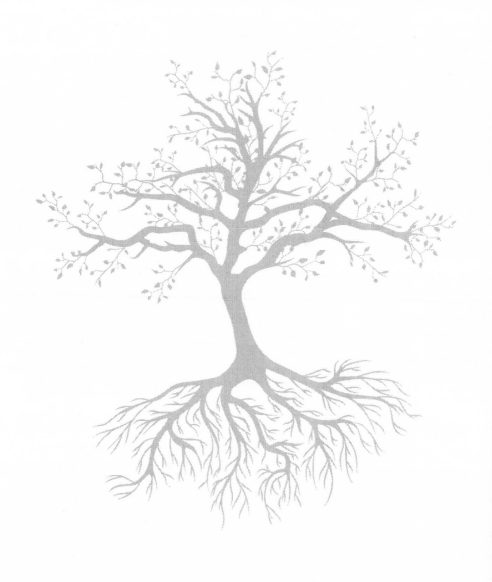

Boundaries Aren't All About Pleasing

Day 21

Be wise in the way you act toward outsiders. Make the most of every opportunity.
Let your conversations be always full of grace, seasoned with salt, so that you
may know how to answer everyone. - Colossians 4:5-6

Why is it so hard to say no? To just simply say, you know I'm sorry but I just can't.
Why are we so quick to please people and quick to make sure we don't upset them?
As an empath, boy do I let that worry fester. Since opening up I have struggled with
pleasing others and boundaries.

Going through a pandemic with a small business , I learned really quickly that a
lot of people forget you are human as well. When I allowed so much access to myself,
I started to feel that I was starting to lose my why and purpose. The struggle making
everyone happy cost a load of anxiety.

With boundaries there is a right way and there is also a wrong way. I am guilty of
doing things the wrong way and I continue to learn what is right. But, the thing my
friend is saying is that it's ok to say no. It's ok to have that boundary of what I like to
call my safe zone. And if the fear is losing people, well the truth is why? Those that
truly cherish you will understand and grow with you.

We just have to use a little more sugar and some Mrs. Dash salt-free seasoning
when we apply or respond.

QUESTION: Do you have a hard time saying no?

_____

_____

_____

_____

_____

_____

_____

_____

_____

_____

_____

_____

_____

_____

_____

_____

_____

_____

_____

_____

_____

_____

_____

PRAYER: Lord help me with the fear of pleasing and upsetting others, to be able to set healthy boundaries. Amen

Affirmation to speaking life:

I am me

Quote of the day: boundaries teach people how to treat you, and they teach you how to respect yourself. - Unknown

Song to add to playlist: Relate - For King and Country

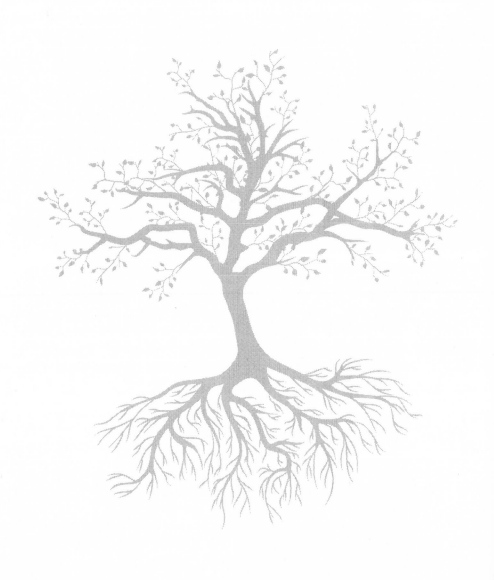

The Fruit of the Spirit

These next 8 days, I take you through each one that I have struggled with. The ones that I cherish. But most importantly each one is part of the foundations that help me with my character. I struggled my whole life with perfection, but one thing I have come to learn is that perfection is nothing, but a lie. Your flaws, your lessons but most importantly the things that make you, you are what the world needs more of. And sometimes it can be a bit much, but its okay. That is where the fruit of the Spirit comes into play.

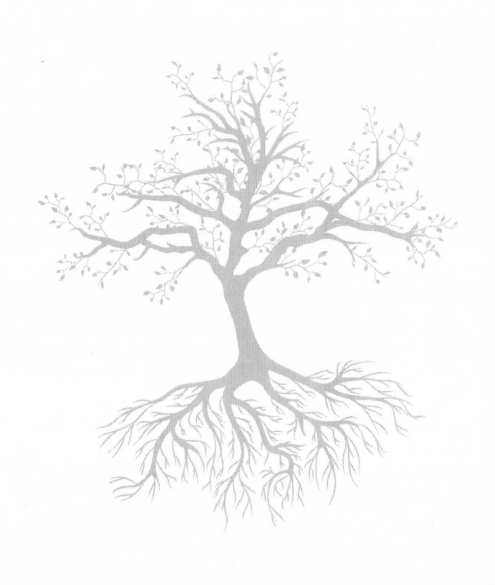

The Simple Joys

Day 22

May the God of hope fill you with all joy and peace as you trust in Him, so that you may overflow with hope by the power of the Holy Spirit. - Romans 15:13

Can you remember a moment of pure simple joy? We get so caught up on the downfalls that happen during the day that we forget to cherish the simple joys Something so simple that when you think about it your smile radiates, or you may laugh until tears run down your face and you can catch your breath and possibly have an accident.

I look back at all the simple joys in my life even during the hard times, those precious simplest moments where for a moment you forget about that trial you are going through and you have that hope and peace that everything will be ok. You see my friends, the joy given to you is what gives you strength to go on. And that is what God loves to sprinkle us with simple moments of joy

One of those simple joys I laugh about now is when I was in kindergarten. I got a role in the play stone soup and I was a protein. I was super excited to be that chicken. I went home and told my mom all about it and a lady at church said oh I can make a costume for you. Those few weeks I went to school excitedly helping my classmates make and paint costumes. It was the night of the show and the lady from church came all excited to hand me mine. as I watched everyone walking as drumsticks and veggies she pulled out a whole chicken custom feathers and all. As the play started and they called out the proteins, here came a big bird hiding behind all the drumsticks and hiding behind the kettle pot. My mom will say, I was the cutest little chicken, I will tell you this is where my butchering of song lyrics and words come from. But looking back all I can do is laugh at this simple joy of a chicken dancing with a bunch of drumsticks. Simple joys oh how I love thee!

QUESTION: What is one simple joy that brings you a good laugh?

PRAYER: Lord, thank you for the simple joys when we go through the hard times, remind me of those simple joys daily for joy is where my hope and strength comes from. Amen

Affirmation to speaking life:

For the joy of the Lord is my strength

Song to add to playlist: Joy - For King & Country

Mindfulness pose: cat cow hold for 5 exhale for 5 repeat for 3

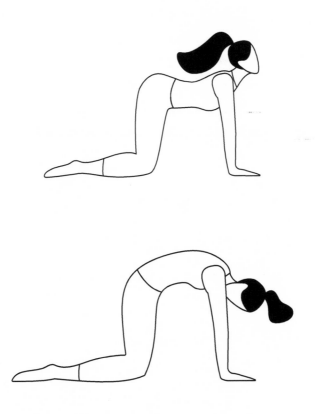

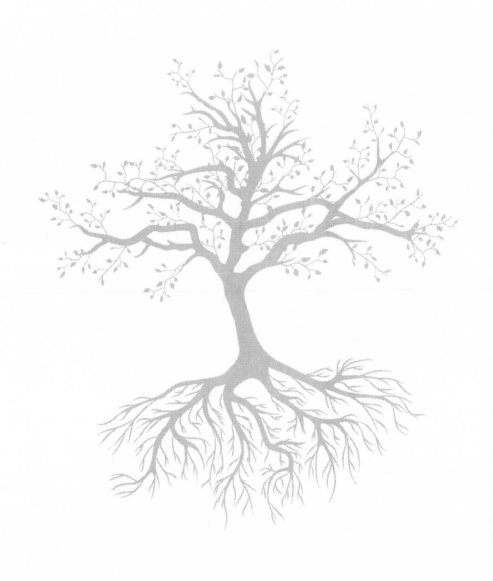

Have Patience

Day 23

But if we hope for what we do not yet have, we wait for it patiently.

- Romans 8:25

Oh, be patient or have patience is where I am either rolling my eyes or I find myself having that toddler meltdown that wants it now! You want me to wait patiently, lol, ok Lord. But, seriously how many times do I try to do things rushing or because I can do it. I will admit, I have moments, usually after a trip to the ER, where I say, "maybe I should have waited."

And I know that God has to have a huge smile on His face as He shakes his head as He sees me again. I can hear Him counting down to the moment I am stomping my feet saying, "Help me Lord!" or I'm praying for forgiveness because I didn't wait. And I am thankful that He doesn't say those famous husband words, "O,h so now you need my help?" I blame my daredevil impatient ways on the book, *The Llittle Engine That Could*. You see, it teaches you to keep going if you don't succeed. Nowhere did it say hold up have patience!

But, what I have learned from my friends is that during the waiting is when the things we are hoping for are being worked on for our good. We just have to be still. I laugh as I write this because at this moment I am having a hard time being patient and being still. And I am back in Sunday school listening to how patience is a virtue. To slow down, when I was booking it out of class. Unfortunately, I say this when Susie cuts me off, whenever I'm trying to drive with Jesus and hit that red light.

So friends, slow down, don't rush it, unless it's a good sale at Bath and Body Works AND you have coupons. But, seriously remember that everything is always done on God's timing, not ours and He already knows the outcome.

QUESTION: What's one thing you are struggling to be patient with?

_____

_____

_____

_____

_____

_____

_____

_____

_____

_____

_____

_____

_____

_____

_____

_____

_____

_____

_____

_____

_____

_____

_____

PRAYER: Lord, help us to be more patient in our everyday lives. Help us to slow down and be still. Even though it's not easy to do. We know what we hope for already has been done for us - Amen

Affirmation to speaking life:

Everything in time. I will be still and know that God has worked everything for my good.

Quote: If God is making you wait, then be prepared to receive more than you asked for. - Unknown

Song to add to playlist: Help is on the Way -TobyMac

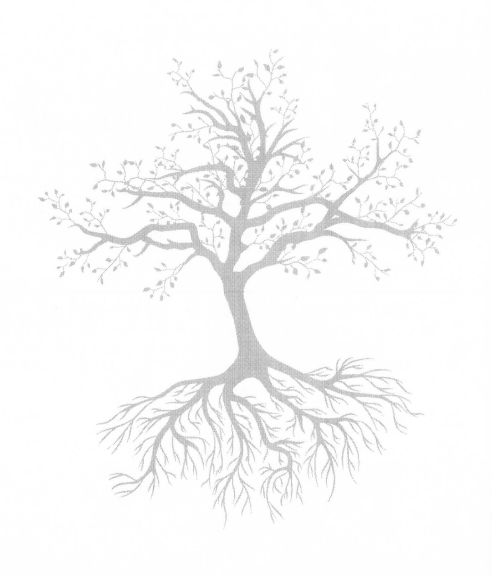

Gentleness

Day 24

To slander no one, to be peaceable and considerate, always gentle towards everyone.

- Titus 3:2

Growing up, I was always taught a gentle word that stirs away anger. Throughout my life, I have forgotten those small little words. To be honest my friends, I know there are a lot of us who have forgotten this too.

You see, we are gentle when it comes to holding that baby, or even packing something fragile. We are gentle when there are people around us. But, when we are alone or responding by text we forget about that gentle word. We are quick to unleash that harsh word with what consumes us at that moment. Instead of waiting with patience for that little moment to pass and respond with gentleness.

I know that I catch myself doing this with my teens or spouse. But, also when I hear something that hurts. The root that I have found that causes this for me is in some of my military upbringing, and that's ok. When I take a moment to walk away or set the phone down and truly process, that's where we can see where that gentle word can be much more than that harsh word ever could. It can build that person up, instead of leaving them feeling so worthless.

QUESTION: How can you be more gentle in your life?

_____

_____

_____

_____

_____

_____

_____

_____

_____

_____

_____

_____

_____

_____

_____

_____

_____

_____

_____

_____

_____

_____

PRAYER: Lord, please help me to be more gentle. Iinstead of trying to make a point and responding with harshness, help me to speak words of wisdom and of life that will bring more peace than strife. Amen

Affirmation to speaking life:

Less criticism, more compassion, more grace, less guilt
- Tai Wo Kafilat

Song to add to playlist: Sing a Song - Third Day

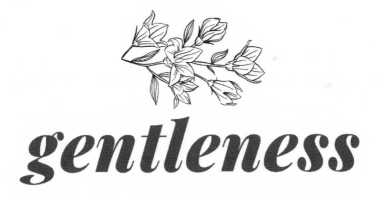

gentleness

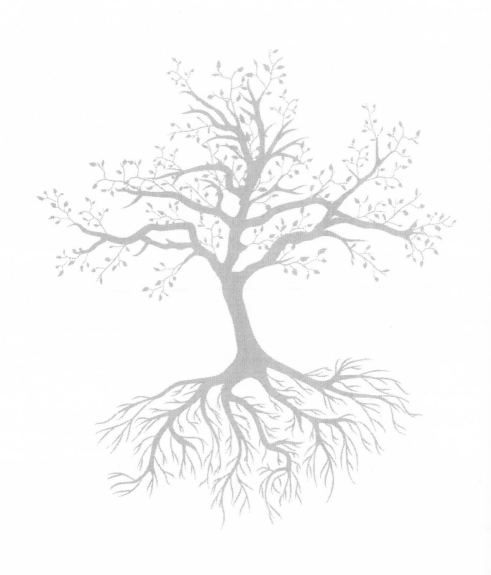

So Simple Yet Free

Day 25

Let kindness and truth show in all that you do

- Proverbs 3:3

Kindness is something so simple, but we often find it so hard to do. Seriously, why is it so hard to be kind these days?

I once responded to someone, when they asked why did you go out of your way to help that person. And I replied, "Because you never know when that may be you in that situation" Sometimes, I believe that it could be Jesus in disguise. I went back to the woman at the well, where she had no idea she was talking to Jesus. I truly believe, if I were to be tested by Jesus or one of His angels this would be the way. Kindness is free! It can be the stepping stone on making someone have a great day or stop them from feeling that they are alone and help them realize that they truly matter.

We have forgotten kindness and are too busy to even realize that those around us may need to be uplifted. I am also guilty, at times, of being so busy and just not being kind. But friends, I challenge you to try a daily act of kindness. It doesn't have to be materialistic, posted on the internet for the world to see! It's just a simple act. A compliment, holding the door, a hug, bringing over dinner to a mama that is just so tired, or just simply praying. The world needs those little seeds of kindness more now than ever, honestly we are all struggling with something.

And let's be real, you never know that the person you are sprinkling that seed of kindness to isn't Jesus in disguise!

QUESTION: If there was one random act of kindness you could do for the day, what would you do? _____

_____

_____

_____

_____

_____

_____

_____

_____

_____

_____

_____

_____

_____

_____

_____

_____

_____

_____

_____

_____

_____

_____

PRAYER: Lord, let me be more like you, to love and be kind. Help me to spread your truth in all my actions. And, when I struggle to be kind, you give me the gentle reminder that it might just be You that I am rude to. Amen

Affirmation to speaking life:

Today I will plant kindness like confetti

Quote: Kindness is a gift pass it on

Song to add to playlist: Humble & Kind - Tim Mcgraw

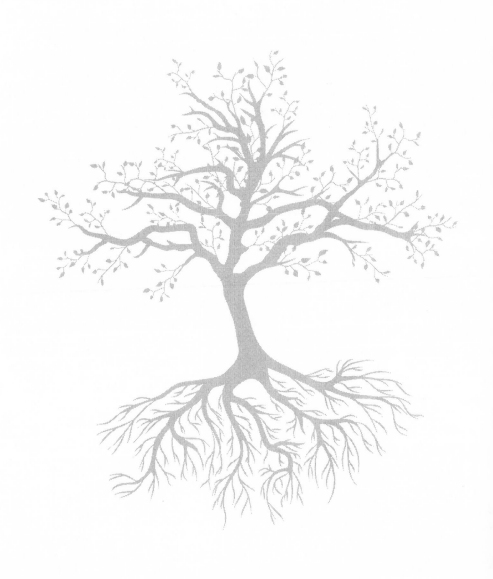

Faith is Like Burpees

Day 26

And God is faithful, He will not let you be tempted beyond what you can bear.
But when you are tempted, He will also provide a way out so that you can endure it.
- 1 Corinthians 10:13

Oh, faith is like that favorite exercise word you hear your trainer say with excitement. "Are you ready for those burpees?!" You give that trainer that side eye, but even as you loathe those burpees, as you go down and jump back up. That right there is just how I describe how faithful God is during the times in my life. Stay with me now.

So when you are down in that storm and feel that you are alone will not make it... With a surge of His grace and mercy, He gives you that power to pop right back up! Now, those burpees are exhausting and you may feel a little queasy. But, when you are finished and you look back, you are amazed that you went through that burner and you are still standing.

How awesome is it that no matter where you are in life, even when you say I don't want to or don't need you to show me. God is right there being faithful and planting more little seeds of faithfulness.

QUESTION: Can you list 3 awesome acts of God's favor and faithfulness ?

PRAYER: Thank you Lord, for always being faithful no matter if it's the super hard times. Even during those great times, you always remain faithful.

Affirmation to speaking life:

I love those faithful burpees :) But no matter what season I am in, God is right there always faithful and guiding me.

Song to add to playlist: Faithful - Elevation Worship

Picture to color

With burpees around it

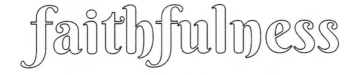

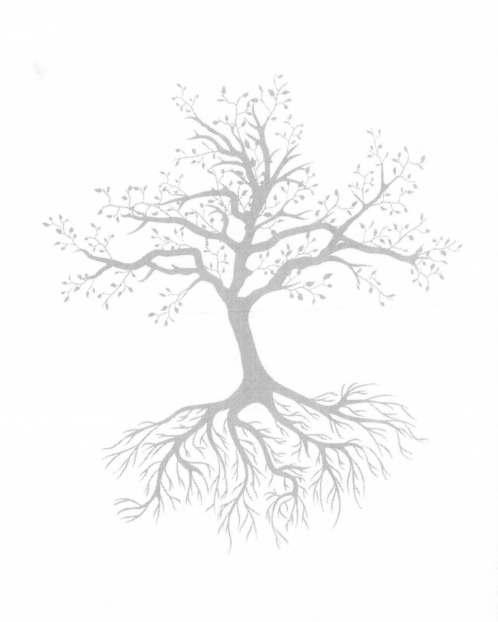

First Moments

Day 27

I have loved you with an everlasting love.

- Jeremiah 31:3

Love has so many meanings to everyone. You have those first "I love yous". You have the love of food and the love of passions. Love is often celebrated and love sometimes ends in heartbreaks. But for me, the moment I learned what true love meant was the moment I became a mom. Each experience of my journey into motherhood was in a different season of my life. But, it was in those first moments I truly understood what and how great love was.

At 18, I was so scared of the type of mom I would be. So many questions ran through that 18 year old mind. But the moment I held my first son, Lucas, and those blue eyes looked into me, I knew I would move mountains for him. And that I would lay my life down with no questions asked. At 23, I was worried if I would have enough love for this second son of mine, but then I saw those old soul gray eyes as Jordan stared at me. I knew I had enough love to give freely and my heart grew even more. And I would do the same for him, as I would for my first. At 34, when the unimaginable happened and I stared into those closed eyes, knowing I would never protect him or show Kellen how much I loved him. I was gently reminded that love knows no bounds and that love is everlasting. And my heart expanded with that everlasting love.

I share this with you, because this is how God reminds me how much he loves us. He loves us freely, will always protect, but also that His love knows no bounds. Just as His love sent his only son to die on the cross for our sins. So, when you question will you ever experience that love, I will tell you, you have it in the palm of your hand. But, also loving someone can be hard and even though we are to love one another. Remember just how much He loves you freely and everlastingly.

And to the ones that say I'm not worthy or capable...Know my friend, you are worthy of all the love! BUT, first you must learn to also love who you truly are.

QUESTION: What is a way you see love? _____

_____

_____

_____

_____

_____

_____

_____

_____

_____

_____

_____

_____

_____

_____

_____

_____

_____

_____

_____

_____

_____

PRAYER: Lord, thank you for loving the hot mess of a person that I am. Thank you for reminding me that I am worthy to be loved and that your love is given so freely.

Affirmation to speaking life:

My love is everlasting

Song to add to playlist: Your Love Never Fails - Jesus Cculture

Mindfulness pose: Knees to chest. Hold yourself for 10 seconds release repeat for 3

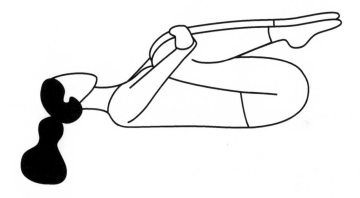

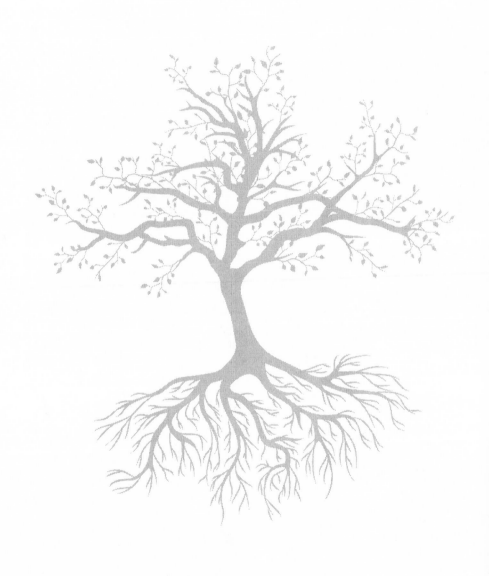

Be Still

Day 28

The peace of God which transcends all understanding will guard your hearts
and your minds in Christ Jesus. - Phillipians 4:7

My dad likes to tell me to seek peace when I'm going through things or when
my temper flares when something has been done. Sometimes, he will remind me
of different stories from the Bible. My mom likes to gently remind me that peace
comes when you trust God and then she send me a scripture or picture she found on
Facebook. I've been blessed with parents that have raised me in faith. But, in my 38
years in this world, I found the moments where I find my peace is where I'm still.

I am mostly still in my refuge sitting on the turf at Rise. Most don't know this but
even as a kid playing soccer, I would sit on the turf or grass before or after each game.
My turf at Rise is where you can find me when I'm there. It's sitting in the quiet
empty gym and taking everything that is happening in. And that is where God shows
up to remind me to be still in this.

If we know that God has whatever we are going through in the palm of his hand
and he gives us peace that surpasses everything, why do we allow our stress to take
over? We let anxiety, doubt and the spirit of fear to take over. Even though we know
that the spirit of fear doesn't come from God, but peace, goodness, grace, mercy and
joy are the root of the things we should hold onto. We just need to be still and not try
to be Bob the builder and try to fix it all.

So, as I rolled my eyes at my dad's long talks he would give me, and look at my
mom like she was crazy, I say this peace comes when we are so still that God shows
up to show us just how mighty He is and how Hhis goodness and grace knows no
bounds.

QUESTION: Do you have a place where you can just be still?

_____

_____

_____

_____

_____

_____

_____

_____

_____

_____

_____

_____

_____

_____

_____

_____

_____

_____

_____

_____

_____

_____

PRAYER: Father, just thank you for showing up when the waves are crashing in on life. You calm those waves and give me peace that always surpasses understanding. Thank you for that gentle reminder that you will never leave me nor forsake us, amen

Affirmation to speaking life:

It's ok to let go and just have peace

Quote: God isn't asking you to figure it out, He's asking you to be still, to trust and as you walk in faith know that He already has it figured out.
- Unknown with a Paola remix

Song to add to playlist: Be Still My Soul - Kari Jobe

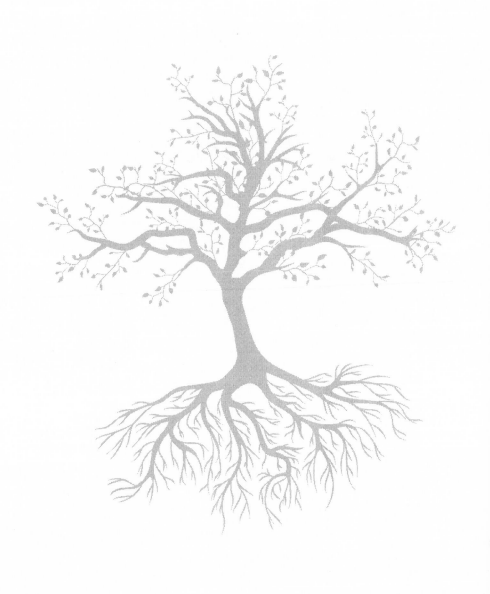

Oh My Goodness...

Day 29

Surely your goodness and love will follow me all the days of my life.

- Psalms 23:6

Everytime I think of the word "goodness", my mind wanders to the Jerry Lee Lewis song, *Goodness Gracious Great Balls of Fire.* Yea, my mind will just rattle to its own beat when I need to focus on the important tasks.

But, this was a great moment when my parents decided to drive cross-country from leaving Panama landing in Florida and driving to our next base in California. We weren't allowed to listen to anything but the Oldies and Christian music. There I was in the back seat of the Camry, between my 3-year old brother and 9-year old sister. And my walkman had just died! So, during one of the hottest days, during a pit stop at a gas station, this was something I decided to sing, at the top of my lungs. Now what does this have to do with God's goodness?

Well, I know I was that typical 13 year old complaining and driving my parents nuts, they allowed me to have my moment of complaining and later provided us with some nice ice cold cherry slurpees. That's how God's goodness is to me. He hears all my complaints, whining, eyerolls and without a single rebuke of frustration. He just shows up blessing me with all these things like that ice cold slurpee on a hot day.

It's amazing what His love can do for you. No matter how much I stumble, falter or try to say, "ummm no God not today." He comes in and says, "Here you go!" And hands over one amazing cherry slurpee! My friend, His goodness, mercy and love is always right there with you. The question is, will you continue complaining about that heat that is going on in your life or will you enjoy that ice cold slurpee?

Affirmation to speaking life:

No matter how much I complain, God still showers me in His goodness

Song to add to playlist: Goodness of God - Bethel Music

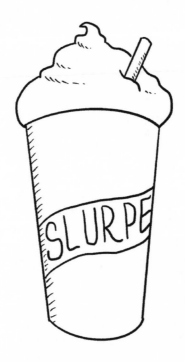

Coming in Like a Wrecking Ball

Day 30

People will be lovers of themselves, lovers of money, boastful, proud, abusive,
disobedient to their parents, ungrateful, unholy, without love, unforgiving,
slanderous without self-control, brutal, not lovers of the good, treacherous, rash,
conceited, lovers of pleasure rather than lovers of God. Having a form of Godliness
but denying its power. Have nothing to do with such people.

2 Timothy 3:1-5

Self-control is the final fruit of the spirit and in truth, the one I struggle with on
a daily basis. This verse describes everything that I have personally struggled with
when I didn't walk hand-in-hand with God. The temptations of this world, the likes
of social media and the desires of the lifestyles that are posted, are some of the hard
things that all of us can say we struggle with.

We shine lights on the things we eat or enjoy, what is purchased, the cars we drive,
the vacations and how much weight we lose and even the famous people we know.
None of that light truly shows the hard work one may have accomplished, the good
and hard times. No, the light is always bright to get likes and feedback.

As I have continued to learn and grow during this past year, and trust me God
has had his work cut out because I am one OCD control freak that stresses out when
things are out of control, He has reminded me, "Does this moment of losing self-
control hurt me? Matter to me? Will it make a difference if it is out of my hands?"
And the answer is a simple no. I just have to remind myself to allow some grace
when I have a moment of losing or struggling with self-control.

Now, on the other side, when you take away my watermelon, THAT does hurt
me. Everyone who knows me knows I have a crazy love for watermelon and zero self
control! I smashed a whole watermelon... You're like, what is this about watermelon?
When we had to shut our business down and my stress level was high my go to

thing to eat was watermelon. I started paying the Kroger price of 8 bucks for that watermelon in March and ended with the July 4th special of $1.99. My addiction to watermelon was so bad my coach removed fruit from my competition plan and when I finally finished my show, the first thing I ate was watermelon. It's hilarious to everyone that knows me. I do not like sweets, drinking or fried food, but when it comes to watermelon or fruit - it is my downfall! I use this to share that we all have our things we struggle with, and sometimes when God removes something out of our life for our good, we may not like it. But, then He brings us something even better and it is just so much sweeter, like that first bite of watermelon!

QUESTION: What is one thing you struggle with self-control?

_____

_____

_____

_____

_____

_____

_____

_____

_____

_____

_____

_____

_____

_____

_____

PRAYER: Lord, thank you for always keeping it real with me as I sometimes struggle with self-control. But thank you for reminding me that your Spirit gave us power, love and self-discipline. When I struggle, remind me of your love and grace. Amen

Affirmation to speaking life:

I am aware and understand my strengths and weaknesses

Mindfulness breathing: Repeat for 3 and release. Inhale through your nose. Hold still do not breathe in or out. Blow out slowly. Hold still once again.

Song to add to playlist: Give Me Self Control - Sovereign Grace

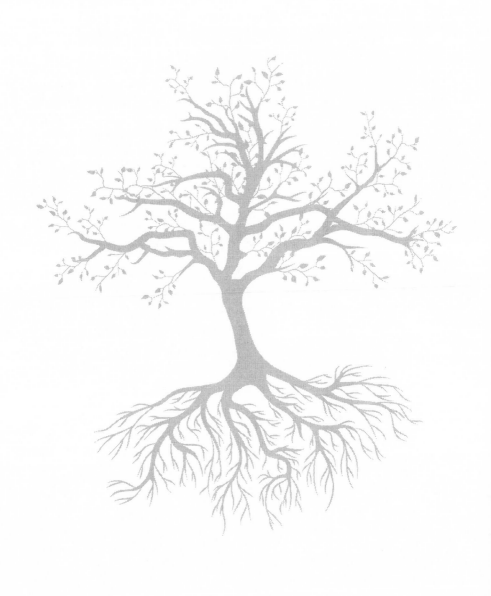

Roots

Day 31

Where you go I will go, and where you stay, I will stay, your people will be my
people and your God my God.

\- Ruth 1:16

Growing up in the military I would always look at the local kids with a slight envy. They had family. They had friends since they could walk. But most importantly, they had roots. My dad had orders every 2 to 3 years. By the time I graduated highschool, I had been to 5 elementary, 2 middle, and 3 high schools. Don't get me wrong, the opportunities and the love of learning new cultures, I loved. But, I always wanted roots.

On this journey I have learned that God has me putting roots all over. The people who come into your life and make an impact on you become rooted in you. When God has you called for a purpose, you are rooted where He plants you. You are there helping others bloom and helping them be able to do the same to others.

When I opened Rise, I was already told that I was there for a season. I just had no idea how short that season would be, and let me tell you how much I miss Rise and its people. But, everytime I go back and see the people, I am reminded of how they are part of my roots.

You see, roots aren't about a town, a home or where you retire. Roots are where you establish your purpose, your impacts, making a difference. It's where you are rooted in strength to help others rise!

QUESTION: Roots can mean so many things. How do you see your roots?

_____

_____

_____

_____

_____

_____

_____

_____

_____

_____

_____

_____

_____

_____

_____

_____

_____

_____

_____

_____

_____

_____

_____

_____

PRAYER: Lord, thank you for establishing me where you needed me to be. Thank you for helping me to be rooted in strength. Help me to love and make the impact you need me to do, in Jesus' name. Amen

Self Affirmation:

I am rooted to rise in strength

Song to add to playlist: Look Up Child - Lauren Daigle

Playlist

Warrior - Hannah Kerr

Beautifully Broken - Plumb

Speak Life - Toby Mac

The Sun is Rising -Britt Nicole

You Say- Lauren Daigle

Another in the Fire- Hillsong

Glorify - Jordan Feliz

Waymaker - Leeland

Overcomer - Mandisa

Counting Every Blessing - Rend Collective

Get Back Up - TobyMac

Thy Will - Hillary Scott

Even If - Mercy me

My Jesus - Anne Wilson

Stars Go Dim - Better

Look What You've Done - Tasha Layton

Women At the Well - Olivia Lane

Great Are You Lord - Casting Crowns

Rescue - Lauren Daigle

O Come to the Altar- Elevation Worship

Relate - For King & Country

Not Backing Down - blanca

Joy - For King & Country

Help is On the Way - TobyMac

Sing a Song- Third Day

Humble & Kind - Tim Mcgraw

Faithful - Elevation Worship

Your Love Never Fails - Jesus Culture

Be Still My Soul - Kari Jobe

Goodness of God - Bethel Music

Give Me Self Control - Sovereign Grace

Look Up child - Lauren Daigle

Thank you so much for being part of my journey. My prayer is that whatever you are facing in life, that you know that you will come through. That you are rooted to rise in strength. That you remember how precious and worthy you are. That you allow yourself grace, even when you may stumble. But, that you keep rising as you continue to trust and walk in faith. And know that He is always with you!

Forever my love,

Paola

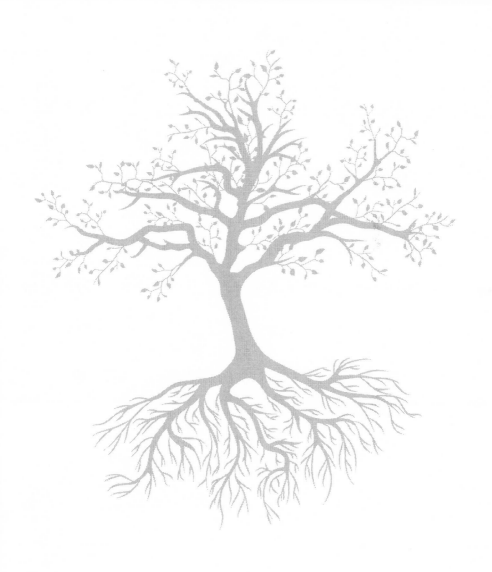